A Caregiver's Guide for Alzheimer's and Dementia

Nine Key Principles

Patricia M. McClure-Chessier, MBA, MPA

Award-winning author of

Losing a Hero to Alzheimer's: The Story of Pearl

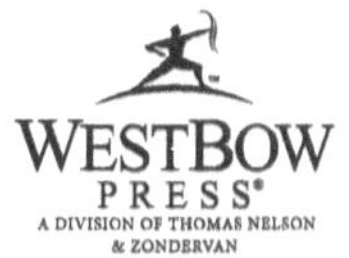

WESTBOW PRESS®
A DIVISION OF THOMAS NELSON
& ZONDERVAN

VATIC Publishing®, LLC

WestBow Press books may be ordered through booksellers or by contacting:

WestBow Press
A Division of Thomas Nelson & Zondervan
1663 Liberty Drive
Bloomington, IN 47403
www.westbowpress.com
1 (866) 928-1240

ISBN: 978-1-9736-4909-0 (sc)
ISBN: 978-1-9736-4910-6 (hc)
ISBN: 978-1-9736-4908-3 (e)

Library of Congress Control Number: 2018914846

Print information available on the last page.

WestBow Press rev. date: 01/22/2019

Patricia's professional and **VERY** personal Insight and experience of "Dealing" with an Alzheimer's/Dementia loved hit on ALL cylinders!!!

Being in the Senior Service Provider Arena for over 18 years as a Non-Medical Home Care Provider, we could of used the 9 Key Principles for my Caregivers and staff to give them more insight and shared experiences. This book will be great in assisting Caregivers and family members in tough situations .

From Key Principle # 1 – Accept & Treasure the Previous Relationship to #9 – Don't Focus on What Others are Not Doing, and those in between should be a **MUST** Primer for ALL of those who are taking care of those with cognitive deficiencies.

Every Family, Health Care Provider, Employer Human Resource Departments, Church Groups and beyond should either get copies of this book and/or have Patricia speak to their Groups to give her insights, personal and professional experiences and support!!

What an Easy Read !!!

Michael Quirk, Publisher,
Seniors Bluebook, LLC
www.seniorsbluebook.com

"The Nine Key Principles offers a solid foundation and unique perspective that empowers caregivers with knowledge and insight to thrive!"

Randy Manns EMT - P/CDP Buds Ambulance,
President of South Suburban IL-COC Association

"Everyone can't be a caregiver, but we can all participate in caregiving."

Patricia M. McClure-Chessier

CONTENTS

Preface

A Caregiver's Guide for Alzheimer's and Dementia equips caregivers to be effective in their role. As a caregiver, you will be assisting your loved one with a range of active daily living skills such as bathing, showering, dressing, grooming, eating, transportation, as well as appointments, management of personal matters, socialization, and more. These principles are designed to give caregivers guidance, avoid pitfalls, and stress the importance of caregivers remaining physically and mentally healthy. Readers will garner hope and understand that while the experience is very challenging, it can also be rewarding. I am confident that if readers follow these nine key principles, they will be better prepared for this tumultuous ride.

In my first book, *Losing a Hero to Alzheimer's: The Story of Pearl,* I share twenty-five years of experience as an educator and health-care professional and my journey as the primary caregiver for my mother who had Alzheimer's. I give a candid depiction of the criticism I faced as a caregiver while other family members watched from the sidelines. After the success and overwhelming response to my story, I wanted to provide readers with a quick reference of some of the errs a caregiver can encounter and offer prevention strategies. This led to the development of *A Caregiver's Guide for Alzheimer's and Dementia.*

Through my travels, I have met several caregivers struggling in their role. This has compelled me to lend my expertise as a caregiver based on my personal and professional experience. To be an effective caregiver requires compassion, love, patience, flexibility, creativity, organization, dependability, and trustworthiness. In this book, I give clear principles and direction on how to specifically handle and interact with the person appropriately and effectively while maintaining your own mental and physical health. There is life after the diagnosis!

Introduction

Alzheimer's has really taken a toll on families all over the world, especially when some of the parties involved refuse to participate in their loved ones' care. I travel frequently to attend and speak at various conferences, expos, best-practice events, media interviews, and book signings across the country. The additional knowledge I have gained from these events, as well as my continued research, has positioned me to meet countless medical professionals and caregivers who have a great deal of questions about my experience. The common thread I've heard repeatedly was that caregivers had little to no support from other relatives. At times, they were under immense stress.

Unfortunately, many did not feel appreciated for being the one who stepped up to meet the needs of their family member.

When people become too focused on what others are not doing, it can exacerbate the situation. After experiencing this firsthand, I have a unique perspective on how to be an effective caregiver with limited support. I often say, "Everybody can't be a caregiver, but we can all participate in caregiving!" It's a blessing to have had the opportunity to be a servant for my mother. It is my privilege and honor to share my perspective and assist others with their role as a caregiver. After reading this book you will have a better perspective on how to be effective as a caregiver.

Alzheimer's or Dementia?

Understanding the Difference

There are several misconceptions about Alzheimer's and dementia. These terms are often used interchangeably when they're actually two different conditions. For example, Alzheimer's is considered a specific disease, while dementia is not. However, the techniques a caregiver will employ during intervention are quite similar for both cases. Alzheimer's disease causes changes in the brain over time, and these changes begin long before any obvious symptoms or lack of cognitive functioning. According to the Alzheimer's Association, our brains have as many as one hundred billion nerve cells, each connecting with others to form communication networks. Scientists believe Alzheimer's disease prevents parts of the cells from functioning properly. When the communication between cells is compromised, problems occur. As damage spreads, cells lose their ability to do their job, which includes storing information, such as memories, and those cells eventually die, causing irreversible and progressive changes to the brain. While it is not the same as dementia, Alzheimer's is the most common cause of dementia among older adults. As the effects of Alzheimer's continues through the brain, it will lead to severe symptoms such as more serious memory loss as well as difficulty speaking, swallowing, walking, and remembering newly learned information.

According to the Alzheimer's Association, dementia is an overall term that describes a wide range of symptoms associated with a decline in memory or thinking skills severe enough to reduce a person's ability to perform active daily living skills (ADLs). Symptoms can vary, but a patient only receives a dementia diagnosis if two or more of these primary mental functions are significantly impaired: memory, communication, judgment/reasoning, the capacity to pay attention, and/or visual acuity. People with dementia can have difficulty with short-term memory, remembering appointments, paying their bills, planning to shop for and/or preparing meals, keeping track of a purse or wallet, or performing everyday tasks. There are many different causes of memory problems. Dementia that is caused by a head injury, stroke, or damage to blood vessels typically is irreversible. Some causes of dementia-like symptoms can be reversed, such as hormone or vitamin imbalances, drugs, alcohol, or depression.

Two common examples of dementia are caused by underactive thyroid and/or deficient levels of vitamin B$_{12}$. People can experience dementia due to Parkinson's disease, Huntington's disease, normal pressure hydrocephalus, and other types of dementia such as vascular dementia and dementia with Lewy bodies, but most cases are due to Alzheimer's disease.

Alzheimer's or dementia can have a tremendous impact on the family dynamic, and the more prepared the family is, the better. Caregivers have to accept a new normal. It may be difficult to accept that the person has a brain disorder or disease, but doing so will enable the caregiver to adapt appropriately and interact with his or her loved one respectfully, both of which are imperative. The nine key principles in the following pages will be a valuable resource, providing integral support to you, the caregiver, as you provide support to your loved one. I will occasionally use these terms interchangeably for the purposes of explaining intervention strategies.

ACCEPT AND TREASURE THE PREVIOUS RELATIONSHIP

One of the hardest things that I had to do was recognize that my mother's behavior changed as her illness progressed. Alzheimer's affects mood as well as personality. Life isn't over after the diagnosis! I had to accept that our roles were reversed, and I was now in a parental role and she in the role of a child. Role reversal is very common when a parent has been diagnosed with Alzheimer's and the adult child is the caregiver. The adult child has to mentally redefine the relationship and take on a new role. This also occurs when a spouse has had to take on the role of a caregiver to a person who was formerly his or her life partner. Due to the brain disease or disorder, you will notice a decline in the person's cognitive level of functioning. Caring for a parent or loved one with Alzheimer's or dementia affects relationships in the family system. Oftentimes, adult children and spouses assume the role of caregiver because of family obligation and love. The caveat is the additional type of relationship can be rewarding. Sometimes I reflect on the changes in our relationship: I was born into this world as my mother's daughter, I later evolved into her friend, and in her final years I became her caregiver. I could never repay my mother for the sacrifices that she made for me, but I was grateful for the opportunity to care for her as an act of my love.

I initially noticed a change in my mother when she started having problems with cooking and handling her finances. She forgot to pay bills and appeared disorganized. My mother had a hard time understanding her personal business matters that she had managed for years with no problem. One of the ten warning signs of Alzheimer's disease is challenges in planning or solving problems. I also recall attempting to have serious conversations with her, the way we had in times past. It was disappointing when she didn't respond the way she used to. Sometimes she couldn't respond at all and would have a blank stare on her face, forcing me to realize my conversation had gone right over her head. I had to acknowledge that her response was going to be different because she processed information differently than before. As a caregiver, I had to let go of the idea of who my mom used to be. I had to accept that my reality was forever changed and keep in mind that hers was too. I realized early on that it was in my best interest to adjust to her reality to avoid being frustrated. It was in my best interest to acknowledge her emotions even if the event wasn't current. There were times that I couldn't always be honest with her. For example, I might not tell her initially that she had a doctor's appointment and just act as though we coincidentally bumped into the physician. This is known as therapeutic fibbing because it's a way of dealing with the anxiety many people with Alzheimer's and other dementias experience in various situations. I had to take heed of the research and use a creative fib to help keep her anxiety at bay, which also inadvertently decreased my stress as her caregiver. This helped in my efforts to participate in my mom's reality. In addition to helping her feel better, engaging in her reality helped me gain her cooperation. Accepting the changes in my mom's behavior forced me to deal with a loss that I wasn't ready to deal with. The fact of the matter is we are never ready to deal with a loss, but we have to. It's a part of life. I felt like I lost my mother and best friend mentally, emotionally, and psychologically— in every way that was not physical. She could no longer give me the emotional support or advice I had grown accustomed to. It was a process, and it took me a while to adjust.

As Alzheimer's progresses, there is an increase in the person's social and emotional detachment. I recall when I had to inform my mother a family member had passed away. Her response was yet another eye-opener for me when she appeared emotionless. She always had a hard time dealing with grief, so her reaction confirmed her emotional detachment. The situations and events that my mother used to find pleasurable and exciting no longer engaged her. She had always been a very sweet and sensitive woman. However, Alzheimer's brought out behaviors that caused her to be emotionless and uncooperative. I had to get used to her being outspoken and saying things that could be hurtful. Mom had lost her filters and no longer carefully considered her words before she spoke. She also had a total disregard for physician's orders, which wasn't like her, and started to refuse to follow her regular special diet and medication regimen. We had to do a lot of coaxing for her to comply, and that was not easy. Prior to Mom being diagnosed with Alzheimer's, she was a stickler for following rules, and this was no longer the case.

Another warning sign of Alzheimer's is changes in mood and personality. The disease may cause the person to be belligerent and combative. My mother started using profanity, which was out of character for her. Additionally, she would display rude and inappropriate behaviors toward me or anyone in authority, including her physician. As time went on, it became more apparent that my mother wasn't the same person. My Pearl was changing, and I had a hard time accepting that, but Alzheimer's is a degenerative brain disease that changes a person's mood and personality, and these changes are inevitable. The caregiver must understand the person is not the same. Both parties are experiencing a loss in different ways. Caregivers should journal their most precious moments with their love one so these memories won't be overshadowed by new, unpleasant experiences. As Alzheimer's progresses, it may be difficult to remember how the person used to be. I found it very helpful in my grieving process to separate Mom as I knew her prior to the disease from the person she had become. It's common for us to remember what happened last. Journaling helps to bottle up those precious memories of what happened best and treasure them for life.

Don't Take It Personally!

8 Ways to Stay Calm

As a caregiver, you have to be the bigger person. Don't take things personally, even when your loved one can't remember important events in your life. Your loved one may no longer remember your birth date or other important dates. Remember, this is just a symptom of Alzheimer's and *not* a deficit in character. Another warning sign of Alzheimer's is memory loss that disrupts life. The main underlying cause of memory loss and confusion is the progressive damage to brain cells caused by the disease. Sometimes your loved one may remember an important date about one person and not the other. Sometimes your loved one may remember something significant about someone whom he or she isn't close to but can't remember something significant about you. There is no rhyme or reason in most cases, so try not to spend a lot of time analyzing why. The human brain is very complicated, and the condition presents other challenges that scientists still cannot fully answer. Someone with Alzheimer's may even lash out at the person taking care of him or her for no apparent reason, and the caregiver may not understand what triggered the behavior. People with Alzheimer's have their own realities that are hard for caregivers to comprehend. They may get upset or angry easily, use bad language, hurl insults, or scream. Your loved one might even throw things or resist your care by pushing or hitting you. This behavior could be a symptom of the disease or just a response to confusion. The person's behavior can be childlike and may mimic a temper tantrum, but it is important to remember that behavior is a form of communication! In some instances, the person may be expressing fear or confusion. We have to ask ourselves what the person is trying to communicate, which should help us not take things personally.

Your loved one will demonstrate behaviors both physically and verbally. Aggressive behaviors may be either verbal or physical, can occur suddenly, could be the result of a frustrating situation, or have no apparent reason at all. While aggression can be very difficult to cope with, it's important for you as the caregiver to understand that your loved one is not behaving this way on purpose. Aggression can be caused by many factors, including physical discomfort, environmental factors, and poor communication.

A lack of physical comfort could lead to aggression if the person is in pain or not getting an adequate amount of rest. It is not uncommon for persons with Alzheimer's or dementia to have problems sleeping or to have an unidentified source of pain (e.g., urinary tract or other infection). They may also experience side effects from medications. Unfortunately, due to their loss of cognitive function, they are often unable to identify or articulate the cause of physical discomfort. Therefore, an expression of physical or verbal aggression may be an indication for you to pay close attention to any potential clues, such as pain during urination. Sometimes my mother was very irritable. I found out later it was due to pain from arthritis in her knees, but she didn't know how to express it. Periodically you have to ask your loved one if he or she is experiencing any pain. Also, we caregivers must keep our eyes and ears open for signs of discomfort.

The environment could also have a negative impact on your loved one, causing overstimulation by loud noises, crowds, or unfamiliar surroundings. This leads to another warning sign, trouble understanding visual images and spatial relationships. People with Alzheimer's may be uncoordinated, experiencing problems with their vision, and have balance and gait deficits. This could put them at risk for falls, which is why the home should be free of clutter and have clear pathways. Unfortunately, the judgment of the person with Alzheimer's is not the same regarding distances and spacing, which is what places him or her at a higher risk for falls. Caregivers should be cautious when changing their loved one's physical environment. I share in *Losing a Hero to Alzheimer's* how I noticed a decline in my mother's condition when we moved to a different home. The person with Alzheimer's may feel lost, which may cause them to exhibit aggression. However, they may be a little bit more alert at certain times of the day, so it is important for the caregiver to identify the best time of day the person functions in and encourage activities and movement during that time in order to avoid accidents. Sometimes people with Alzheimer's experience sundowning, which is a symptom of Alzheimer's and other forms of dementia. It's also called "late day confusion." If someone you care for has dementia, their confusion and/or agitation could get worse late in the afternoon and evening, and in the morning their symptoms may be less pronounced. If the person is experiencing sundowning, the caregiver should do the following: keep a daily routine of when the patient should wake up, sleep, and eat; limit or avoid things that could affect sleep (e.g., radio or television); avoid the person taking a nap within four hours of bedtime; avoid overindulgence in caffeine (especially close to bedtime); and keep things calm in the evening. The routine before bedtime should always be repetitive.

Caregivers should be mindful how they communicate with people who have Alzheimer's or dementia. Convoluted communication could lead to aggression. The caregiver should give simple instructions that are concise and easy to understand. Keep distractions down to a minimum. As caregivers we must be aware of our body postures, facial expressions, and tone of voice more than our actual words. If the caregiver remains calm, it can help the person remain calm. Pay attention to the person's nonverbal cues. Acknowledge their feelings whenever possible. Understanding the person's feelings you are caring for may be more important than the content of the conversation. The caregiver should also be aware of his or her own stress level and emotions when engaging with the loved one. If you are not careful, your stress could invoke anxiety within your loved one, triggering aggressive behaviors or other problems. Having a thorough understanding of what can be a trigger can help prevent the caregiver from taking things personally.

Another warning sign is new problems with words in speaking or writing. People with Alzheimer's may have problems with following along in a conversation and may stop talking in the middle of a sentence. They may struggle with identifying objects and repeat certain questions or gestures. Many misinterpret what they hear. These types of reactions can lead to frustration, misunderstandings, and tension, particularly between the caregiver and the loved one. As the caregiver, try not to show your frustration or anger. Arguing only increases agitation and could potentially make the situation worse. If you find yourself getting upset, take quiet, deep breaths and count silently to ten. Leave the room for a few minutes (only when it's safe!) to gain control of your own emotions.

The Alzheimer's Association recommends the following ways to help the caregiver remain calm, patient, and in control:

1) Remain flexible

2) Respond to the emotion, not the behavior

3) Don't argue or try to convince

4) Use memory aids such as sticky notes, to-do lists, calendars, and alarms

5) Acknowledge requests and respond to them

6) Look for the reasons behind each behavior

7) Consult a physician to identify any causes related to medications or illness

8) Explore various solutions and develop a support system of caregivers and family members who will share their experiences with others

In most cases, a person with Alzheimer's or dementia is in denial. As you know, people with Alzheimer's are unable to reason, rationalize, or comprehend the way they used to. The condition has also caused them to lose the ability to formulate *new* memories. People with Alzheimer's enjoy talking about past memories. Caregivers should allow them to share their memories and reminisce as a way to maintain interaction with them. Memories are also comforting and therapeutic for them. Several people have shared with me during my travels that their loved one treats them the worst or they don't remember who they are. As caregivers, we have to understand that they are not the same person and that is frustrating to them too, so don't take things personally.

Ways the Caregiver Can Avoid Stress

10 Symptoms of Caregiver's Stress

Taking care of someone with Alzheimer's can be a thankless job. Your loved one may not be able to recognize and appreciate the sacrifices you are making. My mother came to live with me and my husband shortly after we got married. It was very challenging because we had someone else to be responsible for. We really didn't have the opportunity to enjoy each other like most newlyweds. When caring for a loved one, it places additional stress on the family system. My husband and I didn't always see eye to eye on certain decisions I made regarding my mother. I was the enforcer because my husband wasn't comfortable with redirecting my mother. If the answer had to be no, he would tell her that she had to speak to me. To hear the word no infuriated her. Most adults do not accept too kindly hearing the word no. The caregiver should avoid using the word no at all costs because it can create a power struggle. The caregiver should create yes opportunities as much as possible. This can be achieved by planning ahead, preparation, and using diversions and distractions when necessary. The role of a caregiver comes with the need to be firm, and there were certain things that I had to stand my ground on because it was in her best interest, such as for safety reasons. However, I discovered a better way of communicating no by learning how to empathize and negotiate with her, which was better for both of us. As caregivers, we have to be flexible and creative. We have to look beyond our loved ones' requests and ask ourselves, *What gratification is my loved one seeking? What can I do that will provide the same fulfillment but with some modifications that will keep my loved one safe?* For example, it may not be safe to take them to the mall but you can take them to a store. Sometimes you may have to pivot or distract the person and get him or her engaged and focused on something else. One key difference between the person with Alzheimer's and the caregiver is that we have the ability to process, remember, and understand the impact of certain decisions.

Caregivers have to be careful with making changes. For example, modernizing a home could create some significant challenges for the person with Alzheimer's.

When we moved from one home to another, it took my mother a long time to adjust to our new home. An acquaintance shared with me how she upgraded her mother's phone from a rotary phone to touch-tone with a caller ID that announced aloud the number of the caller. She later found out that her mother stopped using the telephone because she preferred the rotary phone. I was surprised to learn that every time the caller ID called out numbers, it caused the lady to feel afraid. Someone else shared with me how they upgraded to a modern microwave, and their loved one with Alzheimer's refused to use it. When my mother lived with us, we had a dishwasher, but she refused to use it because she enjoyed washing dishes in the sink. You have to be careful that you are not stopping the person from doing something he or she enjoys. This also allows them to maintain their independence. As caregivers, please consider the impact that any changes in your home will have on your loved one prior to making the change. Even simple changes can complicate your loved one's world and cause them to display aggression. So be careful and minimize change!

Wandering is another behavior that a person with Alzheimer's and dementia can display, which is challenging for the caregiver. In the early stages, they can become disoriented or confused. The person may try to go home, become restless, act nervous or anxious in a crowd, or have a problem locating familiar places like the bathroom. It's not uncommon for people with Alzheimer's and dementia to get lost in a mall. Caregivers, please do not take your loved one to the bathroom and tell him or her to stay right there and you will be back. Your loved one won't remember, and more than likely he or she will start to wander. You can prevent the person from wandering by providing a daily routine, ensuring all basic needs are met, avoiding unfamiliar and crowded places, keeping keys out of sight, using devices that signal when a door is opened, and providing supervision. Caregivers should be more alert at certain times of day. Sometimes the person may be adamant about going to work at a particular time of the day because that is what he or she used to do. Caregivers should also pay attention when loved ones repeatedly state they want to go home. This typically means they're missing something, and the caregiver must dig deeper to find out what it is they're missing and help them to fill the void. Is it a flower or vegetable garden, animals, or collection they're associating with the home that they miss? I experienced my mother wandering, and she was found at an animal shelter. We always had animals, and my mother was missing having animals, so she wandered into what was most familiar to her.

My husband and I had to make many sacrifices. Unfortunately, due to a very limited support system, we couldn't take a long honeymoon. When we went on our honeymoon, my mother's eldest brother and his companion cared for my mom, but that came with a price of anxiety and worry. While on my honeymoon, I thought about my mom constantly. I wondered if she remembered to perform her hygiene, take her medicine and if she was safe. In general, I worried a lot about her starting a fire or leaving the home and getting hurt. When I reflect on my journey, I recognize that I spent a lot of time worrying. I learned as a caregiver that you do the best you can, think one step ahead, and put safety first! After that, you have to turn it over to God and stop worrying. Sometimes safety could mean the next level of care.

Caregivers should be aware of the ten symptoms of caregiver stress as identified by the Alzheimer's Association:

1) Denial about the disease and its effect on the person who has been diagnosed

2) Anger or frustration and a belief that the person is just being stubborn

3) Social withdrawal (e.g., if you don't care about being around your friends, neighbors, and doing activities that you once enjoyed)

4) Anxiety about the future and facing another day

5) Depression that breaks your spirit and causes you not to care

6) Exhaustion that makes it impossible to complete necessary daily tasks

7) Sleeplessness and worrying that the person will fall or wander off

8) Irritability that leads to moodiness and wanting to be left alone

9) Lack of concentration that makes it difficult to perform familiar tasks

10) Health problems that begin to affect the caregiver

Caregivers must take care of themselves first! If you are experiencing high levels of stress, you should speak with your physician. Please take advantage of the various resources available, such as respite care, senior day care, or a companion for the person with Alzheimer's. As a caregiver, you have to acknowledge when you need a break for your own emotional well-being.

PRACTICE PATIENCE

8 Tips for Hygiene Compliance

10 tips for Effective Caregiver Communication

I've learned that understanding comes with education, and patience comes with education. Patience is a word that is used rather loosely, but it takes practice and prayer to implement. When communicating with a person with Alzheimer's, you may feel as if you are interacting with a child. The same patience a parent would use with their child is required as a caregiver. It's important for caregivers to be flexible.

Tasks should be as simple as possible. People with Alzheimer's may forget how to do things that they have done for years, such as laundry. My mother used to do laundry on a regular basis but had a hard time remembering how to operate the washing machine and dryer after the onset of the disease. When I asked my mother if she could clean her bedroom, she appeared very overwhelmed and confused. I had to break the tasks down step-by-step for her. However, there were certain tasks she could no longer do, such as hang her clothes up in the closet. She was no longer able to separate her clothes or fold laundry and place the items where they belonged. Another one of the ten warning signs of Alzheimer's disease is difficulty completing familiar tasks at home, at work, or at leisure. It's important for the person to feel as if he or she is still in control. Loved ones should do as much for themselves as possible to help them maintain their independence; however, Alzheimer's patients should not feel pressured or rushed to do anything. As caregivers, we have to be sensitive to our loved ones' confusion and anxiety. The caregiver should aim for a quiet, calm, reassuring atmosphere and eliminate disturbances. Although we have to adapt to their changing needs, our loved ones will need familiar routines.

Our loved ones should still have choices. However, we must limit the number of choices and ensure all the choices we offer are appropriate. Try to avoid asking direct questions, such as "What do you want for lunch?" It would be more productive to ask, "Would you like pizza or a hamburger for lunch?" Giving them a choice between two viable options can make meal planning easier for the caregiver and less frustrating. As the disease progresses, the person may not be as cooperative with their active daily living skills such as dressing, hygiene, and eating. A lot more patience and flexibility will be required. In *Losing a Hero to Alzheimer's*, I speak about my difficulties in getting my mother to take a shower or bath and change her clothes. As a caregiver, you may have to accept the person will not shower or bathe every day. If a person is used to showering, we should offer a shower, or if they are used to bathing, we should offer a bath. The caregiver should not try to convert the individual, but rather stick with what he or she is most familiar with. People with dementia are often resistant to bathing or showering. They will pretend that they just showered or bathed or may refuse. Unless someone is incontinent, daily bathing is not necessary. Some individuals may have a fear of bathing that could be related to the fear of falling, fear of being cold, loss of dignity in being naked in front of the caregiver, or feeling vulnerable. A sponge bath during the week may be sufficient. The caregiver can use nonrinse soap products to make the process easier. I know this may not be the ideal situation, but the main goal will be accomplished. Here are some tips recommended by the Family Caregiver Alliance the caregiver can use to increase the person's compliance with a bath or shower:

1) Capitalize on an appropriate opportunity to start the undressing process, for example when the person is using the bathroom could be a good time to suggest it.

2) Allow the person to get into the bathtub with only a little water in it and fill the tub after the person is comfortable.

3) Ensure the bathroom is warm

4) Have everything available and ready ahead of time

5) Ensure the water temperature is appropriate

6) Use a warm towel or blanket to wrap the person in after the bath

7) To help prevent falls, the bathroom should have safety measures, device, apparatus like grab bars, nonskid mats, handheld shower head, a shower bench or bath stool to increase safety.

8) The caregiver could play soothing music to give the person a more pleasurable experience.

The person may choose to wear the same clothes every day. Instead of engaging in a confrontation with your loved one, you may have to wash his or her clothes daily or purchase multiple outfits that are exactly the same. The caregiver should buy clothes that are easy to take on and off such as pants or a skirt with an elastic waistband and Velcro shoes. Loose-fitting garments and clothing that is easy to fasten are all strongly encouraged. Clothes should be laid out on the bed in the order in which they will be put on. A person with Alzheimer's or dementia may not dress appropriately for the weather, so it's best to have them choose from preselected outfits that are appropriate for the season. The caregiver should clear out dressers and closets of clothing that is not appropriate. Dirty clothes should be kept in a separate location. Remove dirty clothing from the room to avoid power struggles. As a caregiver, you want to decrease the amount of confrontations as much as you can. Everything is not a crisis, and most tasks don't have to be completed right now. We can become impatient when we are trying to force others to do something in a certain time frame. If it doesn't pose a safety risk, it's not worth the caregiver losing his or her patience and responding inappropriately. The person must believe that he or she still has control and options. The caregiver should be able to see the bigger picture and think outside the box.

We have to be mindful that it may take a little longer for loved ones to navigate through a process, but it's important for them to feel that they are still in control. Sometimes it may not be what you say, but how you say it. If our tone is harsh, it can invoke unnecessary anxiety. Therefore, it is important that we remember these caregivers' tools in establishing good communication:

1) Caregivers should make eye contact to make it clear that they are speaking to their loved ones.

2) Caregivers should speak in a respectful tone with a calm demeanor.

3) Caregivers should speak slowly and use simple words and short sentences.

4) Caregivers should give instructions in a concise manner.

5) Caregivers should be aware of their own body language.

6) Caregivers should be active listeners, get clarification when needed, and validate their loved one's feelings and responses.

7) Caregivers should use distractions when appropriate.

8) Caregivers should avoid engaging in arguments or disagreements.

9) Caregivers should give positive reinforcement (a high-five, a hug, small rewards, etc.) to reinforce the positive behavior.

10) Caregivers should be aware if their loved ones have any deficits regarding their five senses.

It's important for the caregiver to take these tools into consideration when interacting with a person who has Alzheimer's or dementia. Positive communication will solicit better results and build therapeutic rapport.

How to Avoid Awkward Encounters

People with Alzheimer's can feel lost in social settings, and we should try to shield them from feeling awkward. To help the person maintain his or her dignity, people should not treat the person as if he or she is invisible, and conversations should be kept light. I found the best interaction to have with them is being present with them. We should take the lead. Conversations shouldn't be complex. Caregivers should avoid asking difficult questions. For example, "Do you remember°...?" A more appropriate question would be "How are you feeling today?" Ask them "Would you like to paint or draw?" Music is a wonderful activity to keep a person with Alzheimer's connected and engaged. The person should participate in activities where he or she feels comfortable.

Sometimes taking my mother to her doctor appointments was very awkward. The nurse or physician would ask me how my mother was doing in her presence. I didn't feel comfortable discussing my mother's challenges in her presence. To avoid being placed in this awkward situation, I would prepare notes about my mother's status and discretely give them to the nurse and/or doctor. It's unfortunate that medical professionals may not realize the problems that discussions like this in the presence of our loved ones could create. As caregivers, we have to remember that these individuals are adults and are sometimes our elders. Good intentions could be perceived as disrespectful and may make them upset. It can also cause the person not to trust the caregiver. We also have to be careful with the terminology we use. For example, we should avoid using the words "babysitting" or "watching them." These words are associated with children, and phrases like this can be condescending.

Another awkward situation I encountered was when my mother used to pick up items in the store without purchasing them. When my mother and I went to the store, I would have to keep a close eye on her to prevent her from picking up items and placing them in her purse. Unfortunately, she was unaware of what she was doing and the legal ramifications attached to the behavior. To avoid an awkward situation, I didn't allow her to walk through the store without me. Prior to me keeping a close eye on her, my mother placed some unpaid items in her purse unbeknownst to me. The metal detector went off as we were exiting the store. I have to admit, that was one of the most embarrassing moments of my life! When they searched our belongings, my mother had $1.00 socks, headbands, and an assortment of trinkets. She wasn't in need of any of these items, but she picked them up. From that moment on, I kept a close eye on her in the store.

As caregivers, you may find yourself in several awkward situations. It was awkward when we ran into someone we knew. For the people who were unaware of her illness, I would avoid speaking. In situations where I couldn't avoid it, I would say, "Oh, look, Mom, that's ________ from the library." At that point I wouldn't leave my mother's side, and I would take the lead in the conversation. There were a few times that people asked to exchange phone numbers, and I did because I didn't know how to handle it. When they called our home, I would explain to them that my mother wasn't feeling well. As caregivers, we should be thinking one step ahead and try to predict awkward situations to prepare for how we will handle them.

I was very selective about the people I allowed my mother to interact with, and I wanted to make sure the visits went smoothly. Maintaining friendships can sometimes be difficult. Sometimes peers are closer than family members and have very intimate secrets that can complicate the relationship when one of the parties is diagnosed with the disease. As my mother's illness progressed, I think it was very difficult for her close friends to witness. It was challenging for them to redirect her. I remember a lady sharing with me an incident she experienced with her friend of fifty years who had Alzheimer's. One day they attended a party, and her friend was mesmerized with the younger men. This was not because she liked younger men, but because she didn't realize they were both older women now. Her friend had reverted back to them being teenagers. This could have been a very awkward situation if her friend was inappropriate with the younger men. People with Alzheimer's may not be in touch with their age and the present reality, so that alone can create some very awkward situations. Plan and prepare for awkward situations.

Maintaining a Good Quality of Life

Although your loved one has been diagnosed with Alzheimer's, his or her life isn't over. As caregivers, we have to provide them with the best quality of life we can. One of the ways we can do this is to help them maximize their independence. We want them to continue to do as much for themselves as possible. Can they still make a sandwich? Think of ways they can still contribute to the household. When my mother lived with me and my husband, she chose to do all the ironing and laundry folding. Our loved ones still want to feel needed and contribute to the household.

Try to allow the person to participate in social activities or sports events for as long as they can. This leads to the next warning sign, withdrawal from work or social activities. Although they may not be able to keep up with a game, they might still enjoy the atmosphere. My mother enjoyed going to parties and playing bingo. I was able to help her play bingo without drawing too much attention to her challenges, and she enjoyed the socialization. Quality of life is important at every stage. I can recall the backlash I received from family members when I scheduled multiple vacations for my mom. Some family members felt it didn't make sense because she wouldn't remember the vacation. However, I knew how much my mother enjoyed traveling. My father felt it was illogical and said I was wasting money. My mother worked for many years, and it was only fair that she received some benefits from her labor. My mother's condition was also regressing, and I wanted her to see our extended family members before her condition got worse. She couldn't recall all the family members that we visited, but she had a very nice time.

Sometimes you may have to give in to your loved ones' requests. In my book *Losing a Hero to Alzheimer's,* I discuss how my mother enjoyed purchasing cups from the dollar store although we didn't need them. Because I knew this brought my mother happiness, I caved. When her cup collection got full, I would throw them away or give them away and allow her to start her cup collection all over again. Stopping her wasn't worth the additional frustration for me, and it wasn't worth robbing her of the happiness she received from collecting and hoarding cups. As caregivers, we should do whatever we can to add happiness to our loved ones' lives. Think about the joy an infant can bring when you smile, talk baby talk to them and they smile back at you. They don't remember, but it makes both you and the baby feel good at the time. Unlike an infant, the person you are providing care for can benefit if you take photographs of them having fun and show it to them in the days or weeks to come. This will also help to capture memories that you can share with them in the latter stages of their illness, not to mention the precious memories you will have in the years to come.

Diet and exercise produce a good quality of life, and this still holds true for a person with Alzheimer's or dementia. They should be given opportunities to exercise and eat as healthily as they can. For those affected with Alzheimer's, maintaining a good quality of life has a lot to do with minimizing changes. People with Alzheimer's benefit from a stable environment tempered with love, compassion, and patience!

LIVE IN THE MOMENT!

Some of the best moments I had with my mom were living in the moment. People with Alzheimer's will talk about things that happened years ago as if it's current. In the early stages, short-term memory is affected, but as the disease progresses, people will experience a gradual long-term memory loss. One of the ten warning signs of Alzheimer's is confusion with time or place. People with Alzheimer's can lose track of dates, seasons, and passages of time. They have a hard time understanding events that are current or happening in the moment. Therefore, you should live in the moment with them. It's a futile point to tell them that what they're talking about happened in the past. My mother used to bring up old events or discuss people who had passed away over twenty years ago. She would get very emotional, as if the person had just recently died. I learned to focus on her feelings and not facts. I also made sure my facial expressions reflected the emotion she was expressing. People with Alzheimer's can be confused with time and place. Instead of trying to convince the person what he or she believes is inaccurate, the caregiver should focus on the emotions and reassure the loved one that everything will be alright. It's very important for the caregiver not to blow them off or get upset with the emotion their loved one is feeling or expressing. Look for the feelings behind the words, because that is the person's reality.

People with Alzheimer's can exhibit different behaviors that we may have to get used to. We should not throw the bizarre behavior in their faces no matter how abnormal it may appear. For example, my mother used to hoard items in the closet and accuse others of stealing them. This leads us to another warning sign, misplacing things and losing the ability to retrace steps. Rather than arguing with her, I would ask her to help me clean out the closet. I also had to go in her closet on a regular basis to ensure she wasn't hiding food. Perhaps she thought the closet was a refrigerator. When she talked about things from the past, I participated in the conversation. It wasn't worth me chastising her about living in the past or her bizarre behaviors. As caregivers we must live in the moment with them. Living in the moment is a way to acknowledge your loved one's feelings and emotions.

How to Avoid Power Struggles

Power struggles are something most people have experienced with children, but the fact of the matter is they also happen often as a caregiver. Power struggles occur when you make a request of someone else, and it is met with opposition. When a mother asks a child to clean his or her bedroom, a power struggle arises if the child refuses. A power struggle could occur if you ask your loved one with Alzheimer's to brush his or her teeth or take a bath and your loved one resists. We have to be careful how we ask. It should be done in a respectful manner. The caregiver can also make a gesture or give a gentle nudge. For example, "Mom, I will start running your bathwater—let me know when you are ready to get in." The caregiver should phrase the request in a way that the person with Alzheimer's feels he or she is in control. Although the person has Alzheimer's, he or she has the right to make choices and be treated with dignity and respect. Our responsibility as caregivers is to assist and guide them while keeping them safe. It is not our job to control them.

If the person is asking for something that he or she can't have, the caregiver should look beyond the request. As caregivers' we have to meet our loved ones where they're, or somewhere in between, unless the outcome will jeopardize their safety. My mother enjoyed eating fish fillets, and her preference was to eat them every day. Of course, I couldn't allow her to eat them every day because of elevated cholesterol levels; however I had to negotiate with her. We worked together to create a weekly menu, and I had her do it in her own handwriting, which helped her take ownership and feel that she was part of the decision-making process. This is where your creativity as a caregiver will be helpful. As the caregiver, you have to be very mindful of how you communicate. If your response is not appropriate, it can lead to unnecessary power struggles.

Caregivers have to choose their battles wisely. I can recall my mother wanting to wear ankle boots in the summer, and I used to get upset when she wouldn't change her shoes. I had to learn that it wasn't a big deal. After all, people without Alzheimer's wear clothes and shoes that are considered out of season all the time! I had to learn to reason with her and buy jeans/pants long enough that it covered the ankle boots. I recognize that was my own idiosyncrasy because I take pride in being fashionable and wearing clothes and shoes that are conducive to the season. I was also feeling embarrassed and felt that people would judge me for my mother's appearance.

As the disease progresses, people with Alzheimer's struggle with decreased or poor judgment, which is another warning sign. The person's mobility and grooming may also be impacted. It may be uncomfortable and even embarrassing at times for the caregiver, but the caregiver must be bigger than the disease and not worry about what other people think. As caregivers, we might have to dig deep to get to the root of why our loved ones are refusing to do something. For example, if a person is refusing to change his or her clothes, the caregiver should listen to the reason why. It could be for a very good reason. Maybe the person thinks someone will steal the clothes because his or her clothes were stolen in the past. If we take the time to understand, it could make the negotiation a lot easier. As I mentioned earlier, my mother wanted to wear the same clothes every day. Initially I was upset, but then I accepted it and bought her enough of the same outfits for the week. I had to get past my own feelings of shame and guilt. Consistency is very important for people with Alzheimer's, and the fact that she wore the same outfit everyday allowed her to be more independent. She didn't have to depend on me to get her dressed. I had to recognize that my mother's independence was more important than what people might think of me.

Please remember: power struggles can lead to verbal and/or physical aggression from both parties. If you find yourself getting upset and about to lose self-control, take a time-out and adjust your approach. Your loved one is not intentionally trying to upset you. As a caregiver you have to be strong and maintain self-control.

Don't Focus on What Others Are Not Doing

Caregiver's Assessment

Try to not focus on what others are not doing. I learned through my journey that not everyone can be a caregiver. Caregiving requires a lot of nurturing and giving of oneself, and it's okay if a person recognizes that he or she does not have those characteristics. *What happens when no one else is willing to help? It's not fair when you're the only one making the sacrifice. I just don't understand why they won't help; she was a great mother or father!* These are a few of the thoughts that go through caregivers' minds when they are receiving limited or no help. We may frequently think others are not willing to help, but remember to reflect: "Did I *ask* for help?" We should not assume that people will know what we need. We all have strengths and weaknesses. Caregivers will get upset about family members not helping. They'll also get upset when people are helping but not in the ways they think they should. As the caregiver, be fair and remember that we can't have it both ways because everyone is wired differently.

Caregiving is not equal, so don't expect equality. Everyone can participate, but the caregiving may look different. There are many reasons why family members may not help: sometimes family members are in denial, they never had a good relationship with the person, they were mistreated, they can't deal with the emotions and behavior, they have not accepted the person has a brain disorder, they have social issues, or they may have a history of avoiding difficult situations and don't feel confident enough to care for their elder. Sometimes the person has competing demands with their own family. Everyone has strengths and weaknesses, but each person is able to participate in the caregiving role. The word "giving" for some family members may not include personal care but could mean giving of their time to run errands, do the person's laundry, pick up medication, or transport them to doctor appointments. Maybe the caregiver participant can help the caregiver with a responsibility, such as picking up their children. We have to remember that every person's relationship with his or her loved one is different, and this could create unspoken limitations (i.e., unresolved issues). Alzheimer's has a way of exposing things that have been buried for years. Family members shouldn't take it personally when their loved one chooses to live with someone else, or someone else is selected by interested parties. In some cases, that person may become offended and refuse to help because they weren't selected as the primary caregiver. There are several factors that should be considered when deciding with whom the person with Alzheimer's should live. The family should take their loved ones' feelings into consideration. My mother decided to live with me and my husband, but I don't think it was because I was her favorite. I believe it was because she perceived me as being strong, and I was the most stable and dependable at the time when she became sick. Sometimes family members may not be in a position to handle the situation based on the circumstances in their lives at that particular time. The full-time caregiver should provide the person with a safe, stable, loving, clean, and structured environment. The caregiver should be mentally stable and willing and capable of taking care of the person. Every parent knows their children in a different way and is aware of their strengths and weaknesses, so in situations where your loved one is choosing which of their children they prefer to live with, respect their wishes.

The caregiver must be flexible, understanding, and willing to make sacrifices without any resentment. It's not the most ideal situation to split a person who has Alzheimer's between homes. This may increase their confusion. Here is a list of questions the caregiver should review periodically to help assess the status of the person and the relationship:

If there are pets in the home, does the person with Alzheimer's or dementia like animals?

Is my loved one vocalizing that he or she is missing something?

Am I taking things personally?

Am I holding any resentment or unforgiveness?

Does the person with Alzheimer's or dementia have a routine schedule?

Does the person with Alzheimer's or dementia get along with all members of the household?

Is my home a noisy environment? (e.g., small children, crowded with lots of people, frequent visitors/gatherings, loud music)

Am I patient as a caregiver?

Do I have adequate time to devote to my loved one? Am I too busy?

Am I too controlling or domineering as a caregiver?

Do I maintain a safe and clean environment (e.g., clutter-free home and vehicle)

Are my problems affecting my loved one?

Have I made any changes to the environment that could be affecting the individual? (e.g., new/unfamiliar household appliances, rearranged furniture)

Is my loved one living the best quality of life possible?

Caregiving can be a shared responsibility. Although your loved one will not be able to function well in various homes, caregiving is a major responsibility comprised of several different tasks, and everyone who cares about them can and should participate! Who likes to cook? Do laundry? Provide transportation to appointments? Don't force anyone to do anything they're not willing or comfortable doing. Caregivers have to be careful that they're not excluding others because they have it in their minds that no one else can render the service like they can. A caregiver is a very special role that should be done not with resentment but with love, compassion, respect, and patience. It is my hope after reading *A Caregiver's Guide for Alzheimer's and Dementia: 9 Key Principles*, you have gained a better perspective on how to approach your role as a caregiver, be effective, and most importantly identify ways to share the responsibility of caregiving.

A Prayer for the Caregiver

Dear Heavenly Father,

Thank You for the opportunity to be able to take care of _______________________. I count it as a blessing that You chose me to be the caregiver of him/her. God, I ask that You remove any resentment that I may have in my heart. I pray that You will strengthen me and help me to be patient and not take things personally. God, I know that this will be an arduous responsibility, but I can do all things in Christ, who gives me strength! Please give me the physical and emotional strength to provide the best care possible to my loved one. God, continue to replenish me spiritually, so I can display the fruits of the Spirit in my role as a caregiver no matter how exhausted I may become. Help me to display compassion and an unconditional love as I assist with his/her active daily living skills. Help me to embrace every moment in a loving way that is pleasing in Your sight!

I give You all the glory! In Jesus's name I pray! Amen.

A Prayer for My Loved One

Dear Heavenly Father,

Thank You for allowing me to serve in the role of caregiver for ___________________. God, I recognize that, according to Your Word, You are able to heal my loved one fully and completely of illness. However, I also know that You don't make any mistakes, and if it is Your will for my loved one to have this experience, my only obligation is to trust and depend on Your wisdom. Despite the challenges, I am truly blessed to have this opportunity. I thank You for providing me with ample resources and support on my journey. Please increase my capacity to be compassionate, patient, and loving as You guide me through each day. Please remind me to lean on You and to remember that no matter what may come, I am never alone. God, I ask that You help me when I struggle with feeling a lack of appreciation for my labor of love. Please remind me that I am doing this as unto You and not for the emotions that my loved one is no longer able to show. Please help my loved one by giving him/her Your peace and let that peace show through his/her cooperation. Help my loved one to understand and recognize that I am here to help and not to harm. Touch my loved one's mind and help him/her to be as independent as possible for as long as possible. Help me to help my loved one live the best quality of life he/she can. I will remember to give You all the glory and trust that You will never leave or forsake us!

In Jesus's name I pray! Amen.

10 Warning Signs and Symptoms Developed and Published by the Alzheimer's Association

1. Memory loss that disrupts life

2. Challenges in planning or solving problems

3. Difficulty completing familiar tasks at home, at work, or leisure

4. Confusion with time or place

5. Trouble understanding visual images and spatial relationships

6. New problems with words in speaking or writing

7. Misplacing things and losing the ability to retrace steps

8. Decreased or poor judgment

9. Withdrawal from work or social activities

10. Changes in mood and personality

REFERENCES

Alzheimer's Association. "10 Warning Signs," retrieved March 1, 2018, https://www.alz.org/alzheimers-dementia/10_signs.

Alzheimer's Association. "Caregiver's Stress," retrieved March 1, 2018, https://www.alz.org/help-support/caregiving/caregiver-health/caregiver-stress.

Davidson Institute. "The Art of Avoiding Power Struggles with Children," retrieved May 1, 2018, https://www.davidsongifted.org/Search-Database/entry/A10242.

Family Caregiver Alliance: National Center on Aging. "Caregivers Education," retrieved April 1, 2018, https://www.caregiver.org/bathing-dementia.

National Institute on Aging. "Alzheimer's Disease, Aging," retrieved April 1, 2018, https://www.nia.nih.gov/health/alzheimers.

Roth, Erica. Healthline, "7 Tips for Reducing Sundowning," retrieved May 15, 2018, https://www.healthline.com/health/dementia-sundowning.

Reischer, Erica PhD. "7 Simple Strategies to Avoid Power Struggles," retrieved May 1, 2018, https://www.psychologytoday.com/us/blog/what-great-parents-do/201410/7-simple-strategies-avoid-power-struggles.

Sikorski, Pam, Terry Vittone. "How to Avoid Power Struggles," retrieved May 1, 2018, https://www.crisisprevention.com/Blog/April-2016/How-to-Avoid-Power-Struggles.

Acknowledgments

First and foremost, I would like to thank God, who is truly the head of my life, for placing me on this trajectory. I started on my journey twenty-five years ago, when I started working in health care as a caregiver for people with intellectual disabilities and mental illness. This opportunity helped to shape me as a professional caregiver, and I later became a leader and proponent for people with intellectual disabilities, mental illness, and the geriatric population. In the years to follow, I never would have thought that my professional skills would be used on a personal level. When my mother was diagnosed with Alzheimer's, my journey became personal. God allowed me to have both experiences, and I am so fortunate to be able to share it with the world.

I want to thank my husband, Pastor Eric H. Chessier, of Cornerstone Christian Church in Chicago, Illinois, for loving me unconditionally. You walked side by side with me and extended your love to my mother. Thank you for your support and flexibility and allowing me to pursue my passion! Thank you to my older children, Monique, Michael, Michelle, and my son-in-law, Kenny, for your love, support, and encouragement. I love you! Special thank you to my daughter's and junior managers, Erica and Jessica Chessier, for traveling with me across the world and working long hours with me at events. I couldn't have done this without you two! Thank you to my road managers, Ms. Janene E. McClure and godbrother Byron Barnes, for your willingness to travel with me and believing in me! To my friend and sorority sister

Sherell McDearmon, thank you for collaborating with me and your support at various functions. Special thank you to my older sister, Belinda McClure, for your ongoing support! I can always count on you to be in the audience! Thank you to my brilliant colleague Mrs. Olieth Lightbourne, who gave me the wonderful idea to complement my book with prayers. I would also like to thank my editor-in-chief, Mrs. Valerie Thompson-Walker, of Vatic Publishing, LLC for your patience, professionalism, diligence, guidance, and collaboration with the prayer. I look forward to doing other projects with you in the future.

I would like to thank my family and friends for your love, prayers, and ongoing support. I appreciate all the churches, nursing homes, hospitals, and health-care facilities for having me as a speaker/presenter. Additionally, thank you to my readers and the special people who have shared their journeys with me. I have truly been blessed! Last but not least, I would like to thank God for my late parents, Jesse and Ann McClure. You both helped to shape me into the person I am today, and I am forever grateful! May you both rest in peace. To God be the glory for everything He has done!

About the Author

Patricia M. McClure-Chessier is the author of *Losing a Hero to Alzheimer's: The Story of Pearl* and *A Caregiver's Guide for Alzheimer's and Dementia: 9 Key Principles.* Patricia is the wife of pastor/radio host Eric H. Chessier as well as a mother. She has been in the health-care industry for twenty-five years. Her educational accomplishments include a bachelor of arts degree in psychology, a master's degree in business administration, and a master's degree in public administration with a concentration in health-care administration. Throughout her career, Patricia has worked with people with intellectual disabilities and mental illness as well as the geriatric population. Patricia is credited for starting a seniors retirement program for people with intellectual disabilities. Currently, she works as an Healthcare Executive Team Leader at a hospital that is owned by a Fortune 500 company; it is one of the largest health-care facilities in the world. Patricia also serves as an adjunct college professor where she teaches health care and leadership courses.

Patricia's love for writing developed at the tender age of thirteen, when she submitted her first published work to *Ebony Jr.* magazine. While in elementary and high school, she served on the newspaper committee and wrote various articles. Patricia continues to use her skills by writing articles on behavioral health-care topics, aging, and national initiatives for the *Daily Herald* newspaper, Vatic Publishing, LLC, and *Patch* newspaper. She has been featured several times in the *Daily Herald*, *Patch*, *Story Monsters* magazine, and the Authors and Experts website hosted by *Story Monsters* magazine. Patricia is an award-winning author of *Losing a Hero to Alzheimer's: The Story of Pearl*. The book won first place in the aging/senior living category, first place in the relationship category, and an honorable mention in the biography/memoirs category at the 2016 Royal Dragonfly Book Awards. Patricia has done several book signings across the world at Barnes & Noble stores, including California, New Orleans, Florida, Minnesota, and New York. She also has been an exhibitor and presenter at several health-care conferences, schools, libraries, trade shows, churches, special organizations, and expos all over the country, including the Atlanta Ultimate Women's Expo, senior aging expos sponsored by Silver Star Expositions, senior expos by 22nd Century Media, Black American Expo, Jacksonville Senior Expo, and many others. Patricia has received positive feedback for her knowledge and expertise in Alzheimer's and dementia, her authenticity, motivation, inspiration, and her ability to connect with her audience as a speaker.

Patricia has done several nationally syndicated radio interviews on WVON, WSRB, WYCA, and WBGX. Additionally, Patricia has done a few television interviews on *Homekeepers*, which is aired on the Christian Television Network and hosted by Arthelene Rippy. Patricia is a member of Alpha Kappa Alpha sorority, Illinois Continuity of Care Association, American College of Healthcare Executives, and is affiliated with several other service organizations. She is a volunteer with the Alzheimer's Association to help end Alzheimer's disease.

If you're interested in having the award-winning author Patricia M. McClure-Chessier speak or present at your next event, please contact her at pmcclurechessier@yahoo.com.

www.ingramcontent.com/pod-product-compliance
Lightning Source LLC
Chambersburg PA
CBHW031136250726
48655CB00002B/700